To Raheim,

May you continue to live
out your dreams & your
purpose!

Keep living in
your power!
Love 'Mable

Words of Wisdom

from

Women

Around the World

AN INSPIRATIONAL GUIDE & JOURNAL

Curated by *Mable Taplin*

ISBN: 9780578979786

Published by
DiscovHer Life LLC
47 w. Polk
#277
Chicago, IL 60605

Cover and illustrations: Erin Venable & Tamara Robbins

Photographer: Image Makers, Chicago, IL

For information about discounts for bulk purchases, please contact DiscovHer Life LLC at ask@discovher.life or 872-222-9561.

Mable Taplin is available to present the Words of Wisdom From Women Around The World workshop at your live event. For more information or to book Mable as a keynote speaker or workshop facilitator at an event contact DiscovHer Life LLC at 872-222-9561 or email ask@discovher.life. If you are interested in joining the DiscovHer Life International Women's Community sign up at www.discovher.life. Follow Mable on social media: Instagram @Discovher.life Facebook: Discovher Life with Mable Taplin. Twitter @Discovher.life

For my mother, Joanie Girl, because of you I have the courage to be me.

Acknowledgements

To the magnificent women in my village, I am reminded daily of the Bantu term, Ubuntu, which means humanity or I am because we are.
I am ultimately grateful for your unconditional love and support of me. It is because of your openness and vulnerability that women from all over the world will know that they are not alone.

Thank you for sharing you with me and ultimately with the world.

"The true meaning of your life can only be discovered by you!"

–Mable Taplin

Preface

It was Christmas time, 2014 and I was sitting in the middle of my bed crying uncontrollably. It was suppose to be a happy time. I mean Christmas is my favorite time of the year. I love the Christmas traditions of going to pick out a Christmas tree with my family and hosting an annual tree trimming party.

Two thousand fourteen was an amazing year for me professionally. I earned the most money at my corporate job than I ever had. And I raised the most money for the non-profit that I'd founded 3 years earlier.

By many people's standards, I lived a successful life. I had a lovely three-bedroom condo filled with artwork from around the world, a six figure corporate job, and I had a host of family and friends who loved me. But something was terribly wrong. I could not stop crying. When in public, I found myself trying to hide the sadness. I would sometimes run to the bathroom and cry in secret if I could not get home to cry. My bedroom was my safe space. It was the place that I could let my true emotions show.

In my bedroom, sitting in the middle of my bed, I acknowledged the persistent knot that I felt in the pit of my stomach. I allowed myself to let the tears flow. I was finally honest with myself that I was not happy. In fact, I was miserable and depressed. The reality was that I despised my corporate job. I felt like my job was stifling me. I did not feel like I could truly be myself. I was tired of the façade. I was tired of feigning interest in activities that I had absolutely no interest in for the sake of "building relationships" with the team. Cue here, baseball!

I desired to be more creative. I wanted to write books or spend time quilting or crocheting. But there was a voice in my head that kept reminding me that intellectual professional women don't do such things. I was tired of living in the box that other people had put me in since childhood.

This box was created by seemingly innocent commentary that I heard growing up like, "Oh your too smart to like that! You are so good at math and science, do you really need to take that art class. It's ok that you are not that good at writing because people are typically intellects or creatives, but not both. Well how about I wanted to be both! I wanted to express my creativity and my intellect in a way that felt authentic and free to me. But I didn't. I bought into the idea that I could only pursue interest in one thing.

Fast forward to adulthood, I had a packed calendar of all things "intellectual." Reading journal articles and books in my field, networking events, golf outings, etc. I thought these were things that I was "supposed" to do.

I was exhausted from trying to manage all of the expectations of people. Often when I mentioned some of the issues that I was experiencing at work or my displeasure with dating or that I was feeling socially stagnant, it felt like I was complaining or being ungrateful. Thus, I started hiding. I no longer felt safe to express my true feelings. It was as if I was the walking dead.

I was angry with God because I was childless and husbandless! My memory constantly replayed the scriptures in the Bible, "Children are a blessing from God and a woman was created to be a helpmate to a man." I had neither. So I wondered if God was also angry with me. I wondered if I was living my purpose. I questioned my womanhood. I also questioned if my career choice was undermining who I really am.

I craved the space to be who I wanted to be, not whom I thought I should be or had to be in order to survive. It felt like MY SOUL WAS DYING. Therefore, I decided to change my environment and create space to discover myself by embarking on a solo journey around the world. I wanted to experience other cultures and reflect on who I was and who I was becoming.

In 2016, I visited 30 countries and 42 cities on 6 continents. While traveling, I met the most dynamic women. I asked them to share quotes and/or stories that were impactful to them. They shared quotes that they heard from other women, quotes that they say themselves, and even quotes from their fathers. In listening to their stories and hearing their quotes, I saw myself.

Listening to these women helped me to realize that I was not alone. I recognized that women all over the world are faced with similar issues regarding, womanhood, motherhood, and career. However, the ways in which we respond to those issues are shaped by our life experiences, cultures, values, and belief systems.

By sharing their quotes and stories, the women had the opportunity to reflect on their past, pull out the hidden parts of themselves, and celebrate the wisdom that they have gained through shared words of wisdom from other women and men.

One of my favorite quotes is "When you see a nice house, just admire the roof." A Zambian woman, Musonda Mumba, told this quote to me. I met her at a wine vineyard in Constantia Valley, South Africa. After meeting me for just 10 minutes, Musonda invited me to stay at her home in Nairobi, Kenya. When I came to visit, I asked her to share a quote and she shared the above quote. But when she shared the quote, I heard in my spirit, "Comparison is the killer of joy!"

It was an aha moment for me, because I realized that part of my unhappiness and discontentment was that I was comparing myself to other women. I was constantly thinking about where my mother was at my age or what my girlfriends had accomplished at my age or I was striving to be like such and such.

My God! I was twisting myself into a mental pretzel. No wonder I was anxious and depressed. The anxiety and depression was my internal alarm warning me that something was off and that I needed to stop and nurture my soul.

I know first hand that through women sharing wisdom and being vulnerable, other women can be inspired and healed. Thus, I started collecting quotes. These quotes are from women that I've met during my travels, family members, friends, and women that I met virtually. The quotes are the backbone of this inspirational guide. As you read the quotes, I hope that you are inspired to reflect on your own life and gain healing and new perspectives as I have.

Be Encouraged!
Mable Taplin, RN
Chief Encouragement Officer
DiscovHer Life LLC
Johannesburg, South Africa 2017

THE INSPIRATIONAL GUIDE IS ORGANIZED AS SUCH:

The original language that the quote was given is across the top of the page. The English translation is in the middle of the page. At the bottom of the page is my interpretation or the author's interpretation of the quote. The name of the woman who shared the quote and in some cases the person or relative who shared it with her is at the bottom right. The woman's hometown is listed below her name.

You may notice a few quotes that are listed as anonymous. These women chose not to have their names listed for various reasons. However, the home country of the individual is still listed.

There are blank journal pages following each quote so that you can document your thoughts.

INSPIRATION

I

Need to

Seek

Peace

Jn

Reality

*A*nd

Trust

In the

*O*mniscience/*O*mnipresence of God right

Now!

Mable Taplin
Chicago, IL, USA

Maisha sio kutafakari yatakayokuja katika siku za usoni au hata kulia ulichofeli kutimiza miaka ya nyuma; unachohitaji, unacho sasa. denn es fuehlt wie du den Schmerz.

(LANGUAGE: KISWAHILI)

Life does not exist
in
future predictions or past grievances;
all we have for sure is
right here
and
right now.

MEANING:
Live life in the present..

— Lorna Bonareri Nyatome
KISII, KENYA

After reading this quote, I thought about...

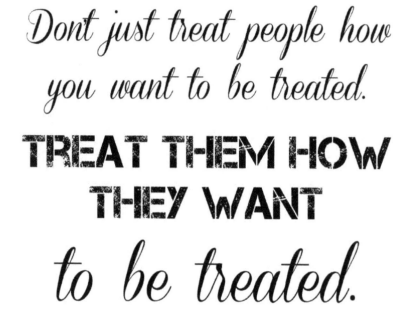

Don't just treat people how you want to be treated. **TREAT THEM HOW THEY WANT** *to be treated.*

MEANING:
When trying to establish a relationship with someone, consider what his or her wants and needs are. Many times, they are different from your own. Considering someone else's needs and wants demonstrates empathy and compassion.

— Toi Esters
LARGO, MD, USA

AFTER READING THIS QUOTE, I THOUGHT ABOUT...

Wer den Pfennig nicht ehrt, ist den Euro nicht wert.
(LANGUAGE: GERMAN)

WE DO NOT HONOR
the pfenning
IT IS NOT WORTH THE
euro,

MEANING:
Take care of the pennies, and the dollars will look after themselves.
Be mindful of the small things and the big things
will take care of themselves.

— Annetta Manson
WORMS, GERMANY

After reading this quote, I thought about...

Hana na wiguri omoyo ni nyumba yoyo ku vandu vosi,
nudake ku dave.
(LANGUAGE: LUHYA-MARAGOLI)

GIVE AND OPEN
your heart
&
house to all,
YOU SHALL
NEVER LACK.

— Sylvia Uluria Commarmond
MBALE-VIHIGA, KENYA

After reading this quote, I thought about...

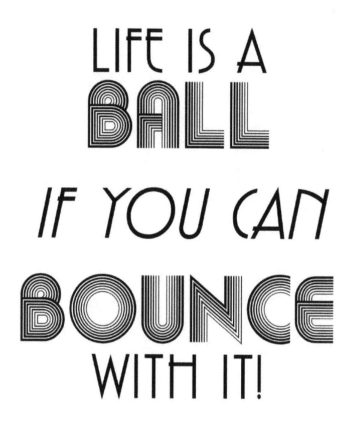

LIFE IS A BALL IF YOU CAN BOUNCE WITH IT!

MEANING:
Life is good no matter what challenges you face. The key to
a good life is learning to go with the flow.

— Darrell Bakeman
CHICAGO, IL, USA

AFTER READING THIS QUOTE, I THOUGHT ABOUT...

THE DRY SKIN
that hangs on
YOUR UPPER LIP
can ONLY *be removed*
by you.

MEANING:
If one is in a pickle or quagmire or tough problem
(e.g. deciding whether to end a marriage/relationship or not)
only THEY can pull the plug, you as a friend or family can just
provide the support and advice. Period.

— Dr. Musunda Mumba
MANSA, ZAMBIA

After reading this quote, I thought about ...

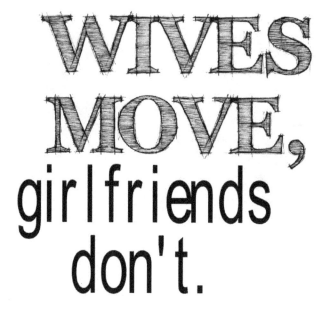

WIVES MOVE, girlfriends don't.

MEANING:
Women may want to consider relocating
for a man when they have commitment.

— Georgette Allen
CHICAGO, IL, USA

After reading this quote, I thought about...

THE WORLD WILL NOT COME

knocking on your door...

YOU HAVE TO GO OUT THERE YOURSELF.

MEANING:
Anything that you want to experience in the world, you have to open yourself up and go seek out the experience.
You have to take action!

—Kathleen Short
YORKSHIRE, UK

After reading this quote, I thought about...

IF YOU'RE
GOING TO HOOT
with the owls
at night

YOU'RE GOING TO HAVE TO SOAR

with the eagles
in the day.

— Anonymous
SYDNEY, AUSTRAILIA

After reading this quote, I thought about...

TEETH AND TONGUE ARE IN THE SAME MOUTH, AND THEY DON'T ALWAYS GET ALONG!

MEANING:
Interpersonal conflict is inevitable. Don't take it personal.

— Elsie Fowler-Watts (mom Fannie Fowler)
CHICAGO, IL, USA

AFTER READING THIS QUOTE, I THOUGHT ABOUT...

BE CAREFUL HOW YOU TREAT PEOPLE.

You never know who will have to give you your

LAST GLASS OF WATER.

MEANING:
You may never know when you will need someone. Therefore, you should treat everyone with dignity and respect.

— Mazie Brodie
PHILADELPHIA, USA

AFTER READING THIS QUOTE, I THOUGHT ABOUT...

Mma ngwana o tshwara thipa ka ſa bogaleng.
(LANGUAGE: SETSWANA)

A MOTHER HOLDS A KNIFE BY THE BLADE.

MEANING:
A mother will do anything in her power
to protect her child from danger!

— Deliwe Radebe
SOWETO, SOUTH AFRICA

After reading this quote, I thought about...

If you *develop a personality* that will cause people to be *happy to see you come* and *sad to see you go,* it will

open doors for you that your looks, your brains, or your *money never could.*

MEANING:
Prioritize learning how to leave positive impressions on the people that you meet.

— Ralphena Dodson
CHICAGO, IL, USA

After reading this quote, I thought about...

HAVE YOUR OWN MONEY!

MEANING:
A woman should always have enough
money to take care of herself.

— Tamberla Perry (Josephine Perry, mother),
CHICAGO, IL, USA

AFTER READING THIS QUOTE, I THOUGHT ABOUT...

Utundu ni adui mkubwa wa uhusiano bora na kujiendelez.
(LANGUAGE: KISWAHILI)

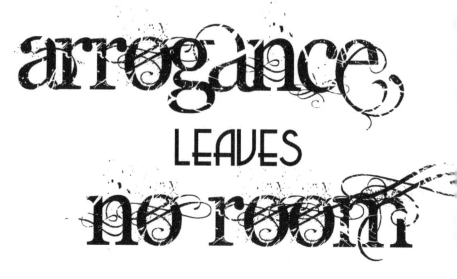

arrogance
LEAVES
no room
FOR INTIMACY OR GROWTH.

MEANING:
When you are filled with pride, it is difficult to form
connections with others.

— Lorna Bonareri Nyatome
KISII, KENYA

AFTER READING THIS QUOTE, I THOUGHT ABOUT...

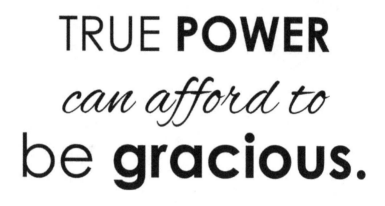

TRUE **POWER**
can afford to
be **gracious.**

— Anonymous
DETROIT, MI, USA

After reading this quote, I thought about...

Umwana ashenda atasha ba nyina ukunaya.
(LANGUAGE: ICHIBEMBA)

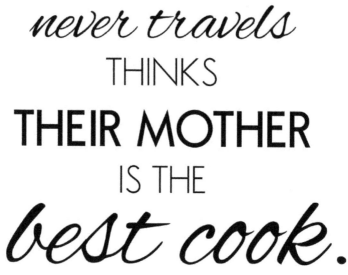

The child that never travels THINKS **THEIR MOTHER** IS THE *best cook.*

MEANING:
The child that is not exposed thinks his parents are the best at everything - basically refering to the narrow-mindedness of being in a limited space. Encourages a person or child for that matter to expand their horizon.

— Dr. Musonda Mumba
MANSA, ZAMBIA

After reading this quote, I thought about...

There are too many devices out here for women to just get married for sex....

You betta

GET MARRIED FOR

some

BENEFITS!

— Mama D
TUCSON, AZ, USA

AFTER READING THIS QUOTE, I THOUGHT ABOUT...

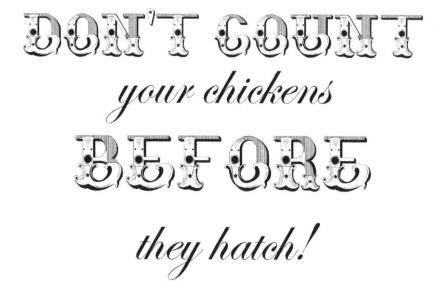

DON'T COUNT
your chickens
BEFORE
they hatch!

MEANING:
Don't use your resources before you have access to them. Ex:
Don't spend your check before you actually cash it!

— Glynda Marioneaux
MEMPHIS, TN, USA

After reading this quote, I thought about...

You are *Beautiful* and *enough* because *God made you!*

MEANING:
Don't use your resources before you have access to them. Ex:
Don't spend your check before you actually cash it!

— Samantha Oliver Mitchell
KLIPTOWN, JOHANNESBURG, SOUTH AFRICA

After reading this quote, I thought about...

Ukwangala kuchila ulupwa.
(LANGUAGE: ICHIBEMBA)

FRIENDSHIP CAN
mean more or
be much more
FOR YOU THAN
family.

—Dr. Musonda Mumba
MANSA, ZAMBIA

After reading this quote, I thought about...

There's a
DEAD CAT
on the line!

— -Belinda Jordan (Ernestine Taylor, Grandmother),
ROSEDALE, MS, USA

After reading this quote, I thought about...

Quaele nie ein Tier aus Scherz, denn es fuehlt wie du den Schmerz.
(LANGUAGE: GERMAN)

NEVER QUARREL A PET OUT OF JEST,

because it feels like you

the pain.

MEANING:
Never torture an animal for fun, it will feel the pain like you do!

— Annetta Manson
WORMS, GERMANY

after reading this quote, i thought about...

Sisterhood
is not dead!

It's one of
the best
"hoods"
to reside in!

— Anonymous,
LOS ANGELES, CA, USA

After reading this quote, I thought about ...

_____

_____

_____

_____

_____

_____

_____

_____

_____

_____

_____

_____

_____

_____

_____

_____

_____

Bez obzira koliko kompliciran i krhki život može dobiti, geografija
moje duše nesumnjivo dokazuje da ljubav nikad nije nemoguća.
(LANGUAGE: CROATIAN)

No matter how complicated and fragile life can get, the geography of

ONE'S SOUL

undoubtedly

PROVES

that LOVE IS *never*

*im*POSSIBLE!

MEANING:
Love is possible regardless of the circumstances.

— Lore Ikovak-Szlapak,
ZEGRAB, CROATIA

After reading this quote, I thought about...

NEVER

let yourself

GET TOO OLD

or too comfortable to put

your foot in a man's chest

DURING SEX!

MEANING:
Don't become complacent in your sexual relationships
with men. Keep it spicy!

—Rose,
USA

AFTER READING THIS QUOTE, I THOUGHT ABOUT...

the day i stop being a child

MY SOUL HAS DIED.

MEANING:
The childlike characteristics of innocence, curiosity, trust, and playfulness are necessary to nurture our souls!

— Trina Beautesansefforte,
DEMOCRATIC REPUBLIC OF CONGO

after reading this quote, i thought about...

You will

UNDERSTAND WOMANHOOD

better when your mother dies.

MEANING:
Our mothers represent unconditional love and support However,
we sometimes judge their decisions harshly.   Loosing your
mother or mother figure may inspire you to reflect on your
life and the influence that your mother may have had on the
woman that you have become.

— Susan Chin,
SINGAPORE

After reading this quote, I thought about...

Kommt Zeit, Kommt Rat.
(LANGUAGE: GERMAN)

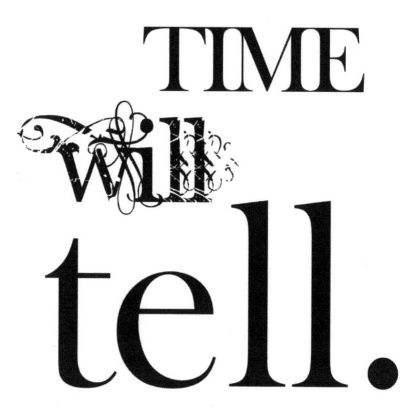

TIME
will
tell.

MEANING:
One's perspective of situations or circumstances
may change as time passes.

— Annetta Manson
WORMS, GERMANY

After reading this quote, I thought about...

Ku n'ganda bakumbwa kofye umutenge.
(LANGUAGE: ICHIBEMBA)

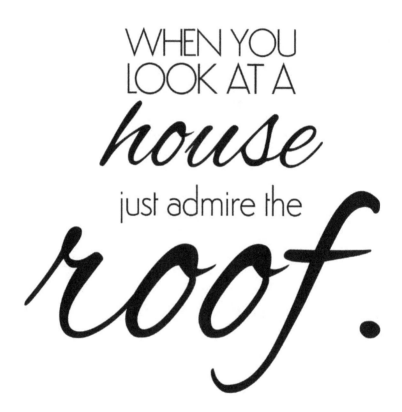

WHEN YOU
LOOK AT A
house
just admire the
roof.

MEANING:
Never admire someone else's life, marriage, relationship, job,
etc. assuming that it is perfect or better than your life. Because
you don't really know what is really happening in their life.

—Dr. Musonda Mumba
MANSA, ZAMBIA

After reading this quote, I thought about...

Xȳā lụ̆m p̄hū̂h̄ȳing pĕn k̄hn k̄hêmk̄hæ̆ng
(LANGUAGE: THAI)

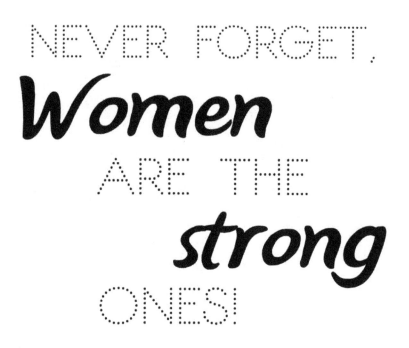

NEVER FORGET, *Women* ARE THE *strong* ONES!

MEANING:
Women are often portrayed as the weaker sex.
This is a declaration that women are strong. Womanhood and strength do co-exist.

—Kotchaphon Wangwon,
CHIANG MAI, THAILAND

After reading this quote, I thought about...

You've got to **know:**
Who you are;
where you are and
what time it is.

— Dr. Sharon Collins (Father, Dr. Ulyssses Duke)
CHICAGO, IL, USA

After reading this quote, I thought about...

Don't you let

NOTHIN' DIE

in your hands!

MEANING:
Make use of your gifts, talents, and ideas. Don't hold on to them until they are no longer viable.

— Terre Holmes, (Great Aunt Helen),
CLEVELAND, OH, USA

After reading this quote, I thought about...

Zuviele Koeche verderben den Brei.
(LANGUAGE: GERMAN)

Too many
Koeche
spoil the pile!

MEANING:
Allowing too much input in a decision or activity can negatively impact the outcome.

— Annetta Manson
WORMS, GERMANY

After reading this quote, I thought about...

YOU GOTTA TEACH PEOPLE HOW TO TREAT YOU.

MEANING:
How you treat yourself and how you respond to how other people treat you will positively or negatively impact how they treat you. Therefore, you are responsible for showing people how you want to be treated.

—Dr. Kenya Grooms
CHICAGO, IL, USA

AFTER READING THIS QUOTE, I THOUGHT ABOUT...

IF YOU HAVE THE

PATH CLEAR

AHEAD OF YOU,

REALIZE AND APPRECIATE THAT

NOT ALL THE PEOPLE

WHO CROSS YOUR PATH

ARE MEANT TO TRAVEL

YOUR LIFE'S JOURNEY

WITH YOU.

MEANING:
Every person that you develop a relationship
with is not meant to be in your life forever.

—Margaret Bunting (sister, Carole Chiloane),
JOHANNESBURG, SOUTH AFRICA

AFTER READING THIS QUOTE, I THOUGHT ABOUT...

una olla vigilada nunca hierve.
(LANGUAGE: SPANISH)

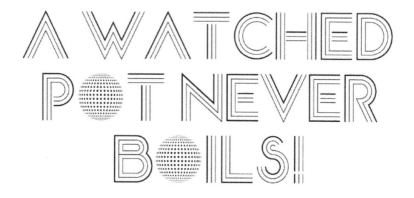

A WATCHED
POT NEVER
BOILS!

MEANING:
Do everything that you know to do for a specific outcome in
life and then let it go! Worrying about the outcome does not
speed up the process.

— Shana Moreno (grandmother, Estelle Moreno),
BAYAMON, PUERTO RICO

AFTER READING THIS QUOTE, I THOUGHT ABOUT...

DON'T TAKE NO WOODEN NICKELS, CUZ THEY DON'T SPEND!

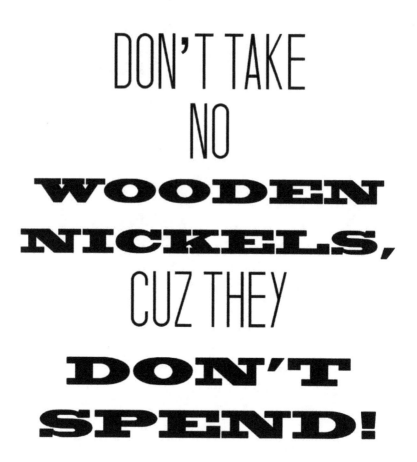

MEANING:
Don't settle for counterfeit things or empty promises, because they will not give you the result that you really want.

— Jeanetta Smith (Annie V. Smith, mother),
ROCKY MOUNTAINS, CO, USA

After reading this quote, I thought about...

Be good.

IF YOU CAN'T BE GOOD,

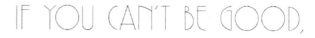

be careful.

IF YOU CAN'T BE CAREFUL,

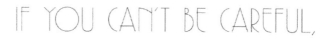

don't do it.

MEANING:
Delight in participating in fun activities, but pay
attention to any potential risks.

— Dr. Ebony Dill (Father, Jimmy Dill Jr.)
CHICAGO, IL, USA

After reading this quote, I thought about...

You can't make a silk purse out of a sows ear!

—Pearlie Taylor,
VANCE, MS, USA

After reading this quote, I thought about...

Ameno maſupa.
(LANGUAGE: ICHIBEMBA)

TEETH ARE
bones, too.

MEANING:
Someone can smile at you with their teeth (ameno) showing
and YET not be genuine at all.

— Dr. Musonda Mumba
MANSA, ZAMBIA

After reading this quote, I thought about...

Kuheshimu uamuzi wa mwenzako, na kumpa nafasi ya kujiamulia mwelekeo wake, kwaonyesha heshima ulio nayo kwake.

(LANGUAGE: KISWAHILI)

HONORing your partner's path and ALLOWing them the SPACE to find their own way sends a clear message of RESPECT.

MEANING:
Recognizing your partner's unique life journey and being patient with their choices is one way to convey that you support them.

— Lorna Bonareri Nyatome,
KISII, KENYA

After reading this quote, I thought about...

The best lesson is a bought lesson, but you don't have to buy them all.

MEANING:

Your personal experience can have an impact on your personal growth, however you can also grow from listening too or observing someone else's experience.

— Joanie Girl
CHICAGO, IL, USA

After reading this quote, I thought about...

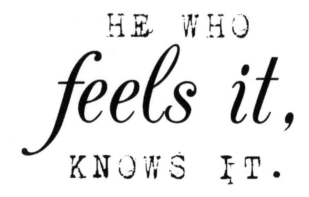

HE WHO *feels it,* KNOWS IT.

MEANING:
Your feelings are true!

—Unknown
LIBERIAN PROVERB

After reading this quote, I thought about...

Keep Livin!

MEANING:
Don't stop pursuing what makes you happy.

— Phyllis Lohar-Singh,
DETROIT, MI, USA

After reading this quote, I thought about...

THE SIGNS BE THERE.

People don't become crazy overnight.

PAY ATTENTION!

—Helen Anderson
CHICAGO, IL, USA

After reading this quote, I thought about

E'erbody who say dey friend,

AIN'T FRIEND!

MEANING:
Everybody who says they are your friend, are not your friend.
Friendship is shown by words and deeds

— Mary Milton
MISSISSIPPI, USA

After reading this quote, I thought about...

Reden ist Silber, Schweigen ist Gold.
(LANGUAGE: GERMAN)

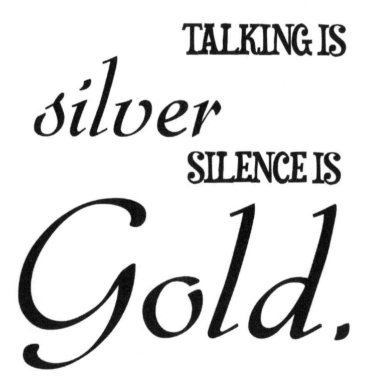

TALKING IS *silver* SILENCE IS *Gold.*

— Annetta Manson
WORMS, GERMANY

After reading this quote, I thought about...

KNOW YOUR WORTH

and except nothing less!

— Saxton Lela,
MONTREAL, QUEBEC CANADA

AFTER READING THIS QUOTE, I THOUGHT ABOUT...

Entre homem e mulher não se mete a colher.
(LANGUAGE: PORTUGESE)

NEVER GET
IN BETWEEN
a husband
and a wife.

— Anonymous
LISBON, PORTUGAL

After reading this quote, I thought about...

Take away
THEIR
EXCUSES!

MEANING:
Always operate with integrity and do your best! Therefore,
alleviating people's motivation and explanations for not
acknowledging or promoting you.

— Dana Todd Pope (Mother, Geneva Todd),
CHICAGO, IL, USA

AFTER READING THIS QUOTE, I THOUGHT ABOUT...

Was du heute kannst besorgen,
das verschiebe night auf morgen.
(LANGUAGE: GERMAN)

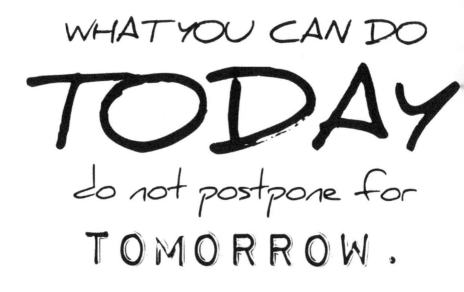

WHAT YOU CAN DO
TODAY
do not postpone for
TOMORROW.

— Annetta Manson
WORMS, GERMANY

After reading this quote, I thought about...

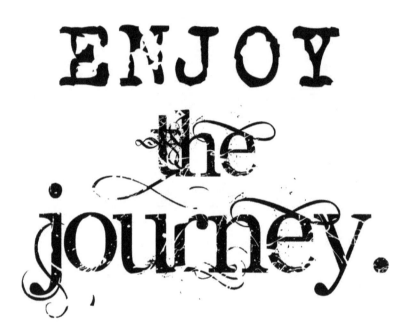

ENJOY the journey.

— Monica Ennis
CHICAGO, IL, USA

After reading this quote, I thought about...

NEVER COMPLAIN
to your family about
YOUR SPOUSE.

YOU'LL FORGIVE YOUR SPOUSE.
Your family
WON'T.

—Donna Wallis
COLORADO SPRINGS, USA

After reading this quote, I thought about...

Lass dir von niemand deine Freude nehmen.
(LANGUAGE: GERMAN)

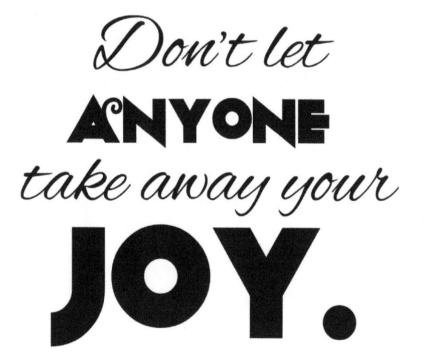

Don't let ANYONE take away your JOY.

— Annetta Manson
WORMS, GERMANY

After reading this quote, I thought about...

IF SOMETHING DOESN'T GET DONE,

it won't be the

end of the world.

IF IT IS THE END OF THE WORLD,

it won't matter

anyway.

— Unknown

After reading this quote, I thought about...

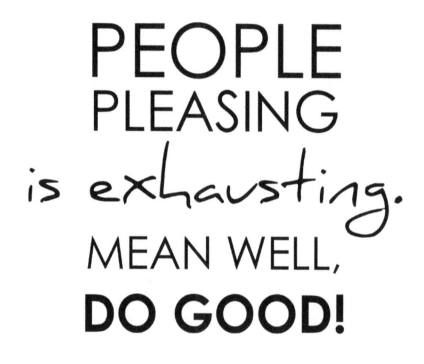

PEOPLE
PLEASING
is exhausting.
MEAN WELL,
DO GOOD!

— Walidah Tureaud (Mother, Gwen Daley)
CHARLESTON, MS, USA

After reading this quote, I thought about...

You have to learn to say

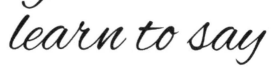

It is the most important word that you will ever use.

— Fran Bell
PHILADELPHIA, PA, USA

After reading this quote, I thought about...

Das wahre Glueck besteht nicht in dem was man empfaengt,
sondern in dem was man gibt.
(LANGUAGE: GERMAN)

true
happiness

does not exist in what
you receive,
but in what you

give.

— Annetta Manson
WORMS, GERMANY

After reading this quote, I thought about…

THE TRUE MEANING

of

LIFE

can only be

discovered

BY YOU.

—Mable Taplin
CHICAGO, IL, USA

AFTER READING THIS QUOTE I THOUGHT ABOUT...

IF A DOG BARKS AT YOU IN THE STREET,

are you going to

BARK BACK?

— Toi Esters
LARGO, MD, USA

After reading this quote, I thought about...

About the Author.

Mable S. Taplin began her career as a licensed Professional Registered Nurse in Chicago, Illinois, and then leveraged her experience to hold healthcare positions in clinical, community, and corporate settings.

Having traveled to over 50 countries, Mable is determined to use her life experience, lessons from her travels, and medical expertise to inspire women all over the word to create their unique path to freedom, passion, and purpose. She facilitates workshops, hosts' retreats, and creates global experiences.

Therefore, she launched DiscovHer Life LLC in 2017. DiscovHer Life LLC is a global lifestyle company that equips women to create their unique path to freedom, passion, and purpose through workshops, online courses, retreats, and global experiences.

As a sought-after author, engaging speaker, coach, and expert on solo travel, Mable empowers women to create fulfilling authentic lives. Mable also enjoys sharing her personal journey and life-enhancing insights on the DiscovHer Life blog and in publications like ESSENCE Magazine.

Mable earned her Master's of Nursing Degree with a focus in Community Health and Leadership from North Park University. She received her Bachelor's of Nursing Degree, Cum Laude, from Howard University. In her spare time, she loves to curl up with a good book, try new recipes inspired by her travels, and dancing in the rain. Above all, Mable still enjoys traveling the globe, forging new friendships, and making children laugh at airports around the world.

Follow Mable on:
Instagram @discovher.life
Facebook: DiscovHer Life with Mable Taplin
Twitter: @DiscovHerlife

Mable loves to hear from you! If you have words of wisdom or would like to share how reading one of the quotes has inspired you, please email wow@discovher.life.

Join the DiscovHer Life community at www.discovher.life

CPSIA information can be obtained
at www.ICGtesting.com
Printed in the USA
LVHW052123131021
700374LV00001B/7